The Magic of Walnuts

Walnuts for Natural Cures And Good Health

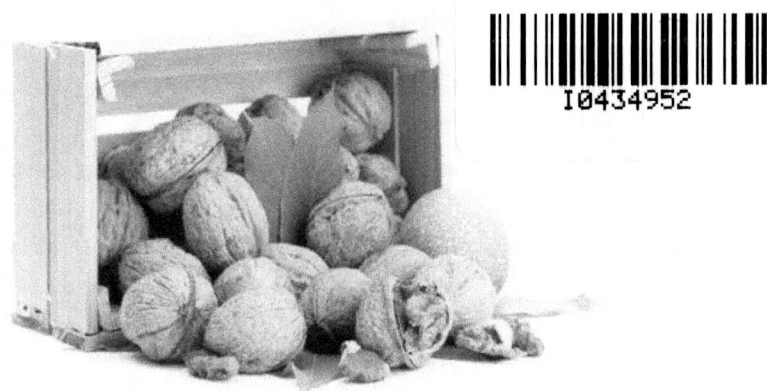

I0434952

Health Learning Series

Dueep Jyot Singh

Mendon Cottage Books

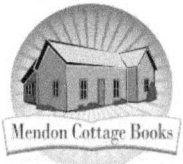

JD-Biz Publishing

Disclaimer

The information is this book is provided for informational purposes only. It is not intended to be used and medical advice or a substitute for proper medical treatment by a qualified health care provider. The information is believed to be accurate as presented based on research by the author.

The contents have not been evaluated by the U.S. Food and Drug Administration or any other Government or Health Organization and the contents in this book are not to be used to treat cure or prevent disease.

The author or publisher is not responsible for the use or safety of any diet, procedure or treatment mentioned in this book. The author or publisher is not responsible for errors or omissions that may exist.

Warning

The Book is for informational purposes only and before taking on any diet, treatment or medical procedure, it is recommended to consult with your primary health care provider.

Our books are available at

1. Amazon.com
2. Barnes and Noble
3. Itunes
4. Kobo
5. Smashwords
6. Google Play Books

Table of Contents

Introduction

Since ancient times, walnuts have been among the most popular – and also the most expensive – of dried fruits available to mankind. If you found yourself in ancient China and happened to be a member of the court of the Emperor, you would show your status by holding a pair of perfectly and symmetrically shaped walnuts. They would be large in size and would be moved around on your palms, while you discuss weighty political matters with the rest of your peers. They would also be rotating and pressing walnuts while arguing the point with you.

The ancient Chinese considered these walnuts pressing their palms to be aids in acupuncture, especially when this pressure promoted the circulation of blood.

If you are in ancient Rome, and were in Julius Caesar's circle, you could perhaps see one of his slaves using red-hot walnut shells as a rather painful depilatory in order to keep Caesar's skin smooth and hairless. Even today, in many parts of the world, burnt and powdered walnut shells are used as a scrub to prevent growth of hair.

A traditional and very politically incorrect old Irish saying says ", *a dog, a woman, a Walnut tree, the more you beat them, the better they be .*" That is definitely not true, because I could not "see" anybody beating a Walnut tree, though, I have been witness to animals and human beings being treated to violence often, and all over the world.

If you were a friend of Leonardo da Vinci in medieval times, it is possible that you may have seen him doing some of his drawings with an ink made up of black walnut husks. Many of these drawings still survive today.

Robin Hood in his mythological adventures always disguised himself by staining his skin with walnut juice obtained from crushed walnuts and walnut husks. This dye was brown in color, and was used for dyeing hair by the ancient Greeks and Romans.

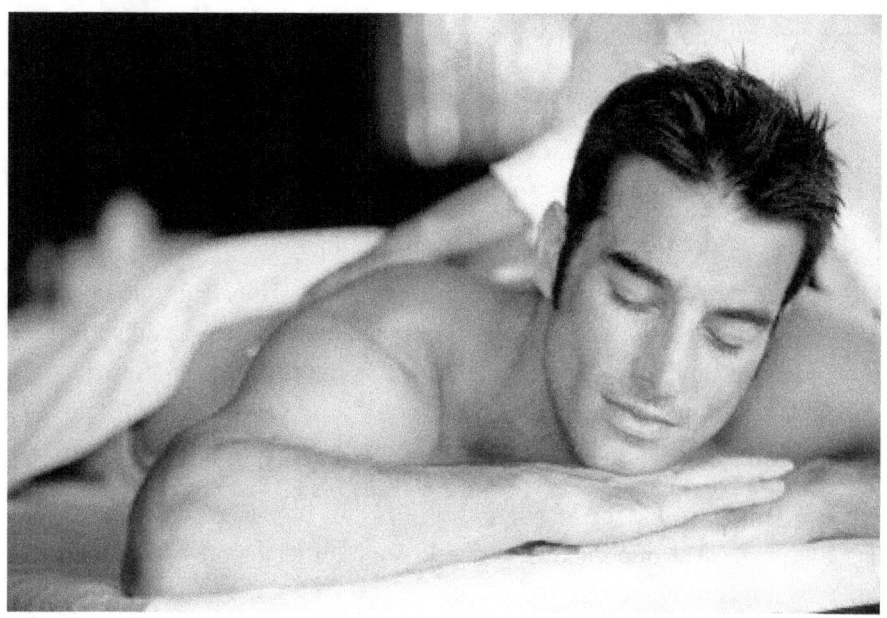

They also used warmed walnut oil for massage purposes. This with almond oil is still being used to aromatherapy to this date.

This nut belongs to a tree of the family Juglandaceae and is called Juglans Regia. The fruit is harvested when it is still green, and pickled. When it ripens fully, it is shelled, and the nut collected as a nutritious and healthy dry fruit.

This not has been long valued as one of the best sources of fatty acids as well as of proteins. In the East, these dry fruits, along with other dried fruits are collected together, and made into winter food by mixing them with molasses and clarified butter, and then pounded. So whenever you feel cold all you have to do is to take a couple of tablespoons full of this warming and proteinaceous powder with hot milk, and consider your system immune from fevers, colds and infections, which are winter related.

After the ripe walnuts are collected, the shells are cracked, so that one can collect the nut. This nut is normally made up of two pieces, and is wrinkled and shaped like a human brain.

This is the reason why, ancient Greek and Egyptian medicine men like Dioscorides considered these walnuts to be extremely good for the brain.

The Magic of Walnuts

According to them, nature had provided visual means in her list of nuts and spices, so that one could just look at them, and see what they were good for. So the kidney shaped cashew nuts were good for the kidney. The almond shape was just like the human eye, so it could be used for keeping the eyes healthy and beautiful. In the same way, walnuts were excellent for the brain.

Most of the time, they were right, because these dry fruits had so many nutrients and good proteins, that they kept the whole system healthy. So people eating almonds would be glad to see an improvement in their eyesight, and would praise Dioscorides for his knowledge. Consider this to be a good case of serendipity, with chance utterances turning out to be true.

A seed kernel is going to being closed in a brown outer seed covering. This has a large number of antioxidants, so do not remove them when you are eating walnuts.

Thanks to the antioxidants in the seed covering, you are not going to get rancid kernels, which would otherwise have occurred as soon as the atmospheric air managed to come in contact with the walnut oil present in the nut.

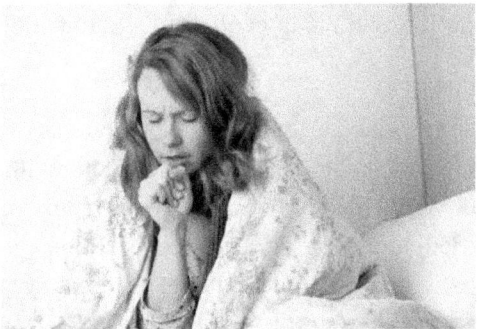

If you have a weak immunity system, add walnuts to your daily diet.

Most popular Walnut Cultivars

The most popular Walnut cultivars cultivated all over the world as well as the varieties which give you the best and sweetest walnuts are the Persian walnut and the black walnut, which is rather rare when compared to the Persian variety. The black walnut is more treasured because of its strong and exotic flavor, but it has characteristics which do not encourage proper and profitable hulling. That is why it is not grown very often commercially, even though it is grown considerably in Northeast America.

Along with the California black walnut, and the Arizona walnut, grown extensively in the USA, especially in the San Joaquin and Sacramento valleys of California, the USA is the third largest producer of walnuts in the world. China leads with 17,000,00 tons annually, followed by Iran producing 450,000 tons annually. The annual production of walnuts in the USA is around 426,000 tons annually, especially the English/Persian variety grown in California and Arizona.

Ukraine, Chile, Turkey, Mexico, India, Romania and France are also among the world's top producers of walnuts.

Apart from these, the more popular Walnut cultivars include Lara, Hartley, Vina, Candler, Hansen, Marbot, Tulare, Ashley, Rita, Valcor and Howard.

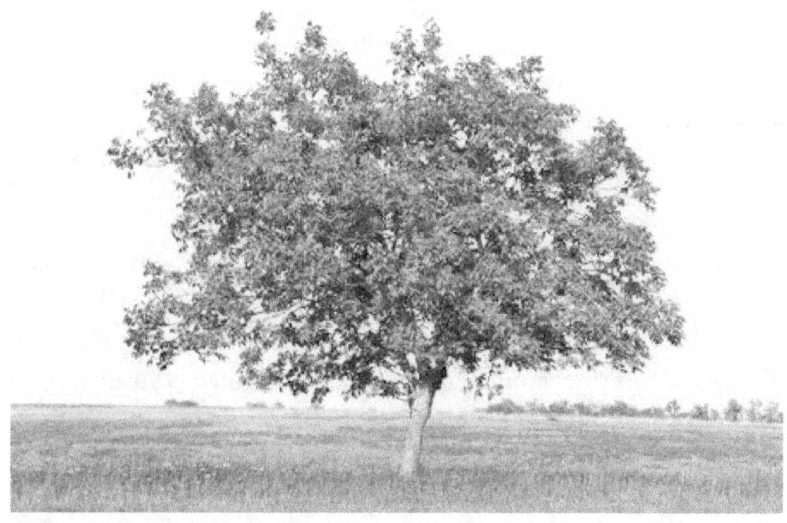

Growing Walnuts

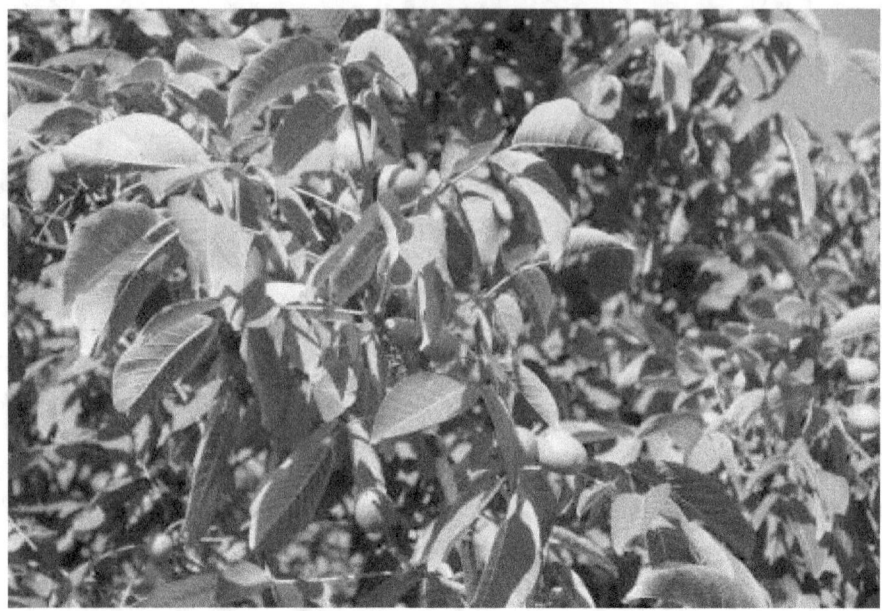

If you think that a walnut tree is going to germinate from those seeds you picked up at the local market, sorry, not gonna happen. You need to get walnut seedlings from a nursery, where they have been grown from healthy cultivars or varieties.

Planning an Orchard full of walnut trees and hoping to hit the market with the produce your your lifetime can be a dream achieved only by those who have patience. It takes about seven years for a Walnut tree to mature enough and start bearing fruit, – it reaches full production strength by the 12th year – but it is going to give you a harvest for the next five generations – i.e. 200 years and more.

That is why the most famous walnut orchards all over the world are family farms, with the knowledge of this plant being handed down from generation to generation. That is because these dedicated farmers know that a little bit of patience and lots of commitment is going to give them a steady harvest of walnuts during their lifetimes.

A healthy full-grown Walnut tree can grow up to 25 m in height, and is thus a popular cannot growing in your garden, along with Apple trees. These trees, which are supposed to originate initially in Mediterranean regions and Persia love the Mediterranean climate. Like many of us humans and cats, they enjoyed plenty of sun. But they do not want it too sunny, and like it as long as the winter temperature does not go below 10°C.

They are going to flourish in a place which is well-drained, well fertilized and deep and with the soil pH value more than 6. They do not like winter frost nor do they like drafts or a windy atmosphere. So plant them in a sheltered area where it is not blow, blow, thou winter wind or even the summer wind.

Some gardeners have found that these plants flourish in soil in which lime and gypsum has been added. Suitable quantities of essential organic nutrients promote the growth of these trees, but that is a given.

Traditionally, 940 walnut trees are planted per hectare, giving each tree a place of 16 into 16 m. These trees are planted in early spring, so that the best growth happens before the onset of the summer. Proper mulching is essential to give you a good tree growth result.

The best seedlings use as rootstock are black walnut, on which other stocks are grafted. If the soil is wet, black walnut is used, but if the soil is well-drained, you can use the English/Persian walnut variety as rootstock.

Wind pollination works best for Walnuts, so you may want to plant complimentary plant varieties which are going to assist with proper and systematic pollination. Walnut trees, just like Apple trees have long been favorites in gardens, because they are shady and long lasting. So you may also want to plant this shade tree in your garden.

The only problem with growing walnuts is that they secrete some chemicals into the soil, which does not promote the growth of ordinary fruit and vegetables in the vicinity. So, a Walnut tree is not going to grow very well in a fruit, flower or vegetable garden and vice versa.

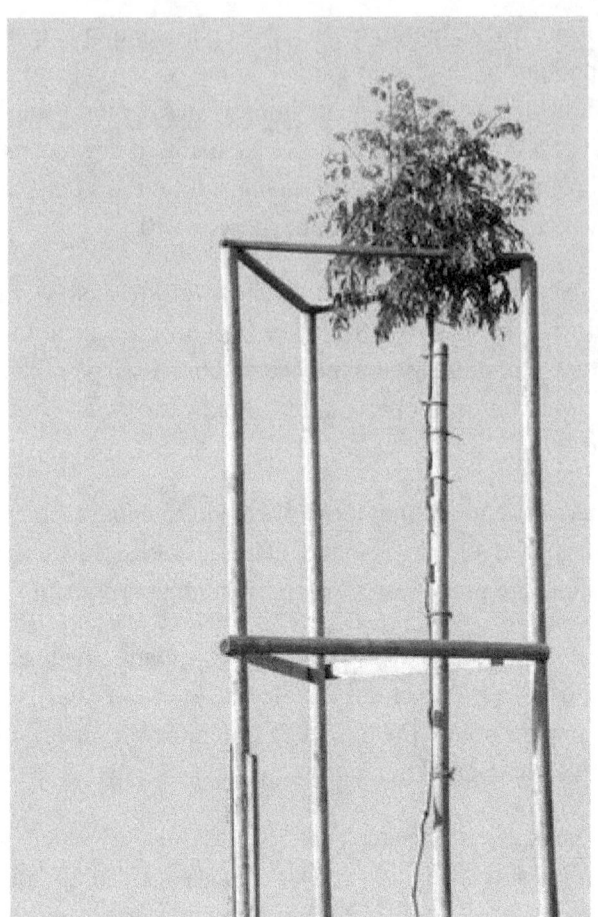

Harvesting

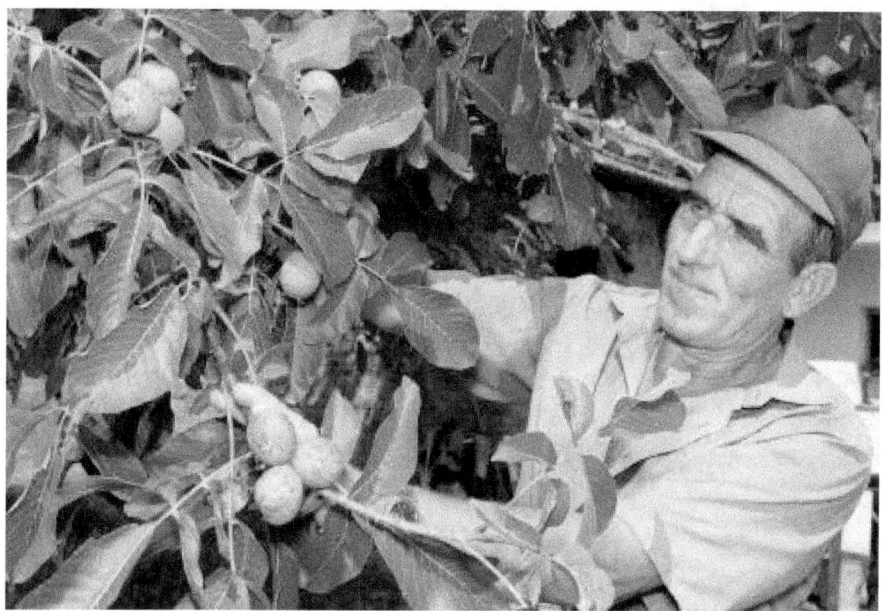

Crops are best harvested with the tree reaches the age of seven and more. The dry green hull of the fruit is going to split and that is why you can shake the fruit right off the tree onto the ground of the orchard. Well, this I believe is what the old Irish meant – a Walnut tree, the more you beat it the better it be. But that is the case for any fruit bearing tree, especially during the harvest season.

Harvesting normally takes place in early spring, which means April depending on the climate, location and the type of the Walnut tree being grown.

Nowadays people use mechanical shakers to shake and shake the walnut tree until every piece of fruit breaks free. These walnuts are then carefully gathered into rows from where they can be collected and taken to the cleaning shed.

The processing process is normally done by removing the outer husk which is green in color. You can either do this by hand, as it was done traditionally millenniums ago. Or if you have thousands and thousands of fruit to be dehusked in a limited period of time, you can use a commercial mechanical huller.

This is the machine which is normally being used by commercial walnut growers in California. The nut is then dehydrated through mechanical systems which use dry air to leave just 8% of the required moisture level in the nut. This drying process is going to take about two – three weeks, depending on the moisture level present in the nuts.

This means that this moisture is just enough to protect the nut from deteriorating and spoiling. It is also going to preserve the quality of the nut.

Walnuts, unlike a number of other dry fruit are going to deteriorate the moment you shell them. That is the reason why like many almond varieties, they are marketed in their shells.

Storing Walnuts

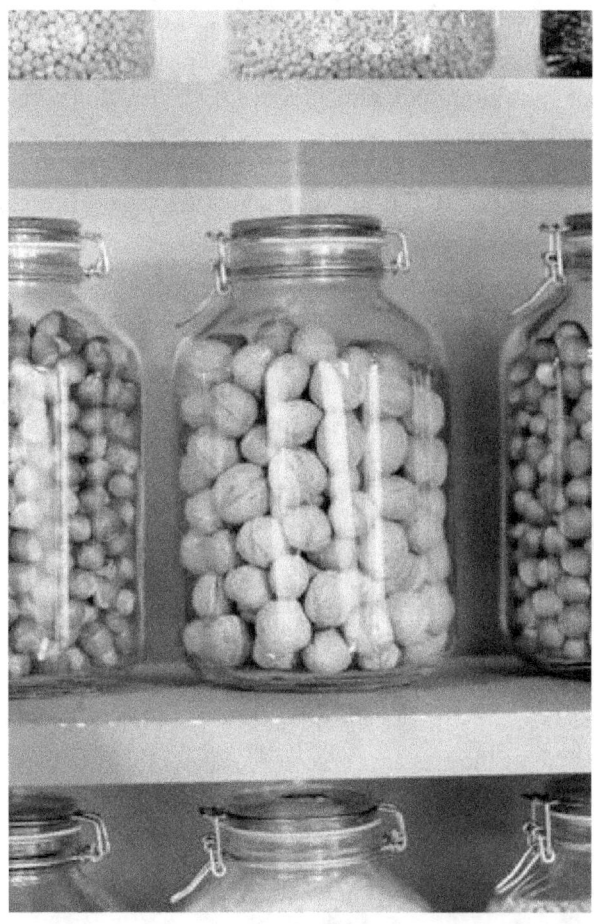

If you have grown walnuts for home use, you may have dried them in racks. Walnuts grown for commercial use are normally dried by mechanical methods. These have to be stored in storages which are totally moisture free. Otherwise, these nuts are going to be subject to fungal infections and insect infestations.

Any batch of these walnuts which have been infested with fungal mold should immediately be discarded. That is because the infestation is potentially dangerous, because of the production of aflatoxin, which is a very strong carcinogen.

Home storage and commercial storage is done best in temperatures ranging from -3 – 0°C. However, there are many parts of the world where such optimum temperatures are not present in refrigerating systems. That is why they store these nuts at temperatures below 20°C, and with a very low humidity to prevent fungal infections.

Any temperature above 30°C is going to cause the rapid disintegration of the nut and the whole batch will need to be discarded. If the humidity is about 75%, you are going to have fungal mold growth on the nuts. So low-temperature and low humidity is best for storing the walnuts.

I would suggest putting them in an airtight container and placing them in your refrigerator. Leave the cover off for the first 24 hours, so that any sort of moisture does not accumulate on the sides of the container. Then put the airtight lid on. Do not use a plastic bag for storing. I just do not trust them, even if you are using them for storing things in the refrigerator.

Raw walnuts, which have been freshly harvested are going to be the best flavored and colored fruit which are going to give you the most nutrients. So if you are around a place where some of your friends are harvesting walnuts off the farm, go on a weekend and share in the harvesting. And then request some of the freshly harvested walnuts in lieu of a days pay. If your friend is a sportsman, he is going to pay you in walnuts.

Nutritive Value of Walnuts

Walnuts, like other dry fruits are extremely nutritional. They are rich in omega-3, vitamins B6, B1, B2, B3 and B5 protein, fats, dietary fiber and amino acids. That is why they are so excellent a food item, when eaten whole, pickled, candied, dried, roasted, and raw.

A cornflakes or muesli breakfast is going to give you more energy, if it has chopped walnuts added to the fruit and milk. This is the reason why walnuts are so well-liked as toppings, and also ingredients of cakes and Christmas puddings.

Walnut oil like salad oil is excellent for dressing, but it is not used for cooking because the smoke point is low.

Walnut Granola

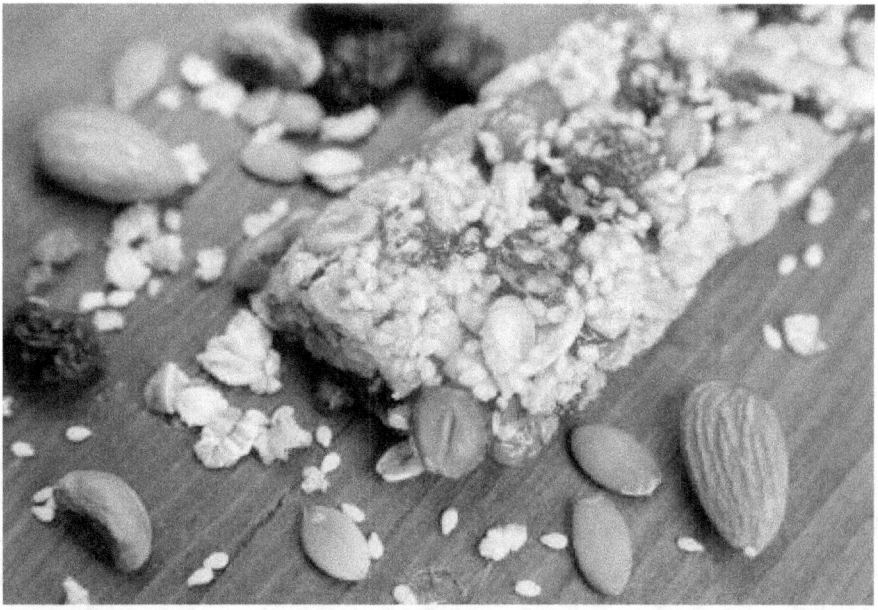

This nutritious breakfast is for all those of us who want a crunchy snack early in the morning. Best accompanied with yogurt as a topping sprinkled on your favorite yogurt dish.

For this you need 4 cups of oats. Use the quick cooking variety. Instant oats will not do. 2 cups of bran for dietary fiber, 1 ½ cups of walnuts, chopped, half a cup of honey, 1 ½ cups of dry fruit like raisins, sultanas, dates, dried apples, dried cranberries, dried blueberries and any other dry fruit on which you can get your hands.

Preheat your oven to 300°F. Stir the bran, oats, and walnuts in a large container or bowl.

Combine the vanilla and honey in a bowl, which can be microwaved. Microwave for about 20 seconds, until the mixture is runny. Pour this runny mixture on your mixed dry ingredients. Toss or mix with a fork, so that all the dry ingredients are coated well.

Spread this in a baking pan evenly and allow to bake for 30 minutes until golden at 300°F. Remember to stir two – three times for even baking.

This granola is going to get crisper, as it cools. Now stir in all the other dried fruit and raisins and store in an airtight glass jar.

You can make this granola in 40 minutes and enjoy as a brunch, breakfast, or just energy giving snack.

Walnuts to Cure You

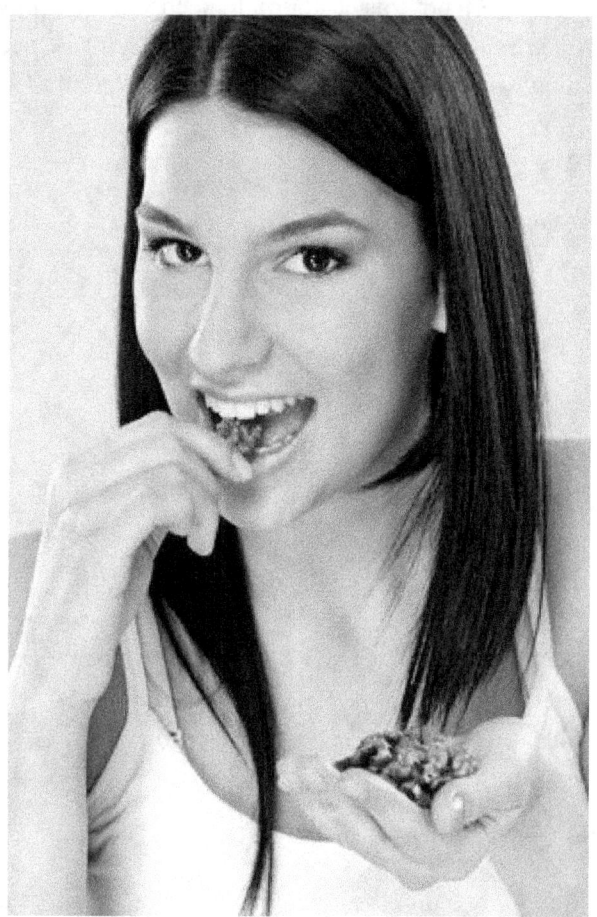

According to ancient medicinal traditions, walnuts are considered to be "hot" in Constitution. That is why they are eaten less in summer and more in winter. You just needed to eat a fistful of walnuts, every day in the winter and keep healthy for the rest of your life. That was if you were of a normally healthy Constitution.

Otherwise, you could eat just those amounts of walnuts, which you would digest properly in a day.

If you have been eating too many walnuts, counteract their heat producing properties by munching on apples and lemons.

The Magic of Walnuts

Walnuts for Constipation

Walnuts are about as effective as castor oil to keep your system working properly. If you are suffering from chronic constipation, you need to eat. Walnut nuts along with raisins. This is going to cure you of this problem.

Pain in Joints

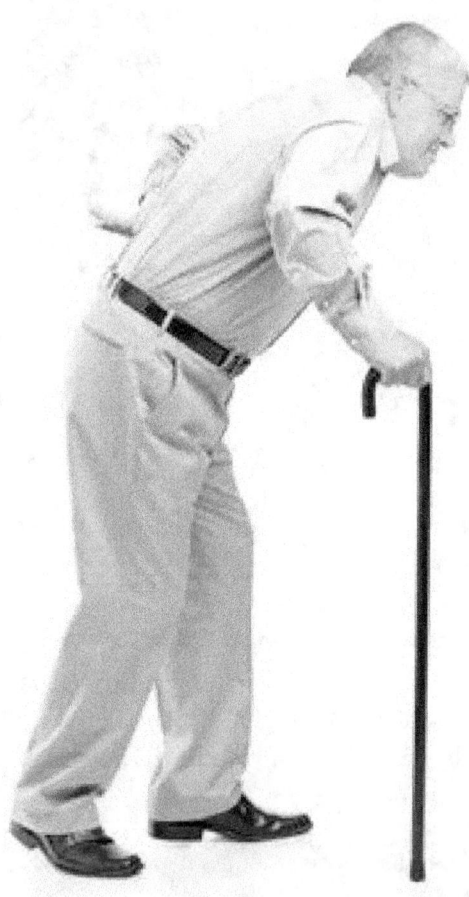

Walnuts are excellent for giving old people healthy and fit

If you are suffering from joint pain, especially new to old age or due to weather, make sure that you increase the intake of walnuts. Joint pain normally attacks people whose lifestyle is sedentary, and also people who are prey to obesity and old age.

These symptoms can be seen by a sharp pain in your joints, swelling, redness, a little feverishness, lethargy and weakness, heaviness in the joints, difficulty in moving about and also chronic constipation. Try adding fresh fruit, green vegetables, fresh fruit juice, mung sprouts and fenugreek to your diet too, along with walnuts.

Do not eat or drink tea, coffee, food items made out of processed flour like pastries, cakes, ice cream, sour items, sugar, cold drinks, tobacco, and such other toxin producing items.

Eat five walnuts first thing in the morning on an empty stomach, chewing them properly.

Walnuts are extremely good for gout. This is because it is considered to be the best natural remedy to clean blood and heal gout. Try this remedy, if you are suffering from swollen toes, which are painful.

Grind some walnuts with a little bit of warm oil and apply on the painful area. Wait until they are dry, and then foment that area with a hot cloth foment. This is going to alleviate the pain.

Traditional Toothpaste Out Of Walnuts

As a child, living in a very old cosmopolitan city, somewhere in the South of India, I was fascinated by the traditional herbs and medicines used to make beauty recipes and other natural items for beautification. One traditional toothpaste made by the grandmothers of these aristocratic ladies, came all the way from Iran and Persia. It used the ground up of roasted bones to make toothpastes. Talk about getting calcium, as well as an abrasive powder.

But we do not have to go to that extent to get our toothpaste. Take 50 g each of Walnut and almond shells and burn them in a frying pan. That is done easily, just keep stirring them on heat until they burn up completely. Then add 5 g of medicinal/edible camphor, 5 g of roasted alum, one gram of peppermint and grind them together.

Mix all these ingredients together and place in a glass jar. Brush your teeth with this traditional powder. This is excellent to cure any sort of disease in your gums and in your teeth. Also, they bring back the shine to your smile, while keeping your teeth really white.

Now there are two types of camphor which are available in the market today. The synthetic camphor is definitely not edible. The edible camphor is, and is called **pachchai karpooram. I have not found it anywhere else in the world, except in the South of India with more information on this particular website.**

http://www.wildturmeric.net/2014/08/benefits-uses-of-camphor-for-skin-hair-acne.html

A pinch of this edible camphor is used to add aroma to sweetmeats.

Here are some sites online where you can find edible camphor.

http://www.herbalveda.co.uk/index.php?dispatch=products.view&product_id=30535

Walnuts for Improving Your Memory

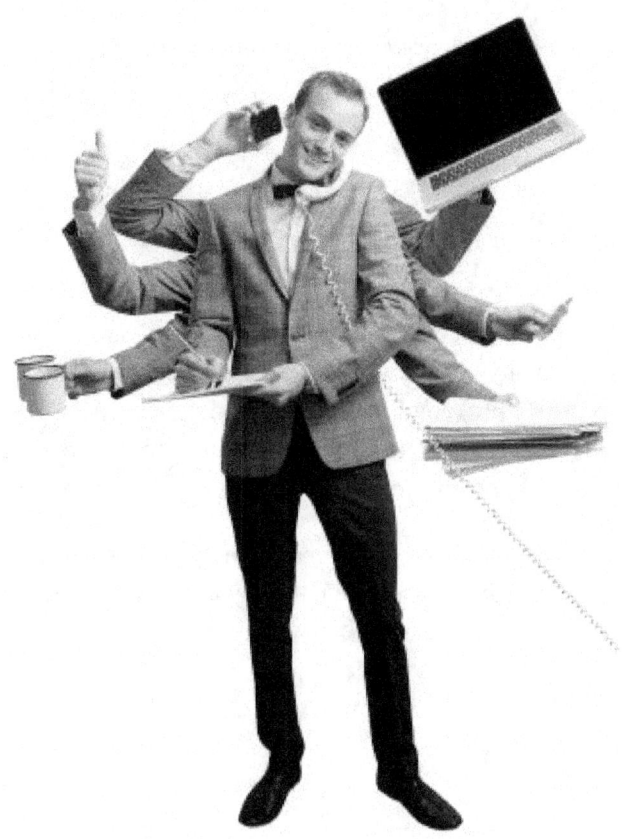

Busy, busy, busy life eh? Add walnuts to your daily diet.

Walnuts have long been considered to be one of the most important of brain foods down the ages, because they are supposed to be memory aiders and boosters, and help to improve your concentration.

There is a scientific reason for this belief. Walnuts have large quantities of omega-3 in them. This is an essential fatty acid which cannot be manufactured by the body and has to be obtained through natural food items like nuts and fish. 25 g of walnuts are going to give you 90% of these essential fats required to keep your system working in a healthy fashion.

The Magic of Walnuts

The brain cells have an outer layer which is almost always composed of fatty tissue. To make sure that there is no lessening of this fat needed to keep your brain working in a proper manner, you need natural omega-3.

Children who have been deprived of this fat because of their diet are soon going to find themselves with slow concentration power and a low memory. They are also going to suffer from insomnia.

That is why, in traditional times, children were given almonds and walnuts. Every evening, with milk, these dry fruit were fed to them to keep them healthy, physically and mentally.

In the same manner old people were also given these dry fruit, so that they did not suffer from any chances of dementia, as they grew older. Also, loss of memory would be prevented when five walnuts were eaten with every meal, every day over a long term. It meant that when they reached their 70s and 80s, they would not start to forget.

Also walnuts were considered to be an extremely good way in which people who suffered from depression or mental fatigue could find their health returning and their mental strength growing better.

Natural Walnut Tune-up Tonic

Here is the natural traditional breakfast tune-up tonic, which has long been used in the East as well as in the Middle East where dry fruits can be found in abundance.

For this you will need to breakfast on this healthy Walnut and other mixed food breakfast which is not only nutritious, but it is also healthy. It prevents constipation, allows you to use sleep well, and also increases your memory and concentration power. In fact, in the East, it was considered to be one of the beauty and attractiveness enhancers, because of the walnuts and the almonds and raisins.

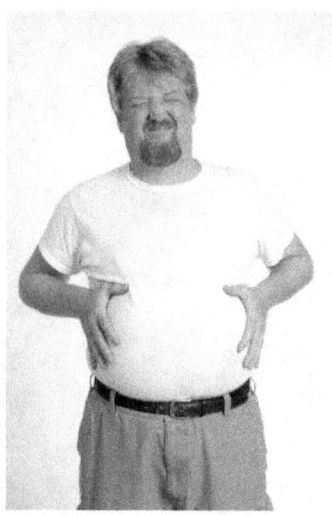

Walnuts in your daily diet help prevent constipation

The reason is quite clear. Keep eating healthy dry fruit every day, and you are going to find a visible change in your health. A healthy person is always attractive, when compared with a sickly looking person. So not only is this human psychology, but this is also good sense.

For this breakfast food – you need three Walnut kernels, half a teaspoonful of poppy seeds, 2 tablespoons full of wheat grain, seven raisins, seven almonds and wash them. Soak them in just enough of water, which is going to be absorbed when you leave them overnight.

The next morning put 250 g of milk on the boil. Add this mixture to the milk and allow to boil five – seven times. Now heat one tablespoonful of ghee, seven black peppercorns, and two cloves in your wok. When the ghee – which is also known as clarified butter or butter oil in the West, is really hot, switch off the heat and add the milk to it.

Now add rock sugar and honey, according to your taste and breakfast off the most energy giving breakfast thought up for you by the ancients.

Now what is clarified butter?

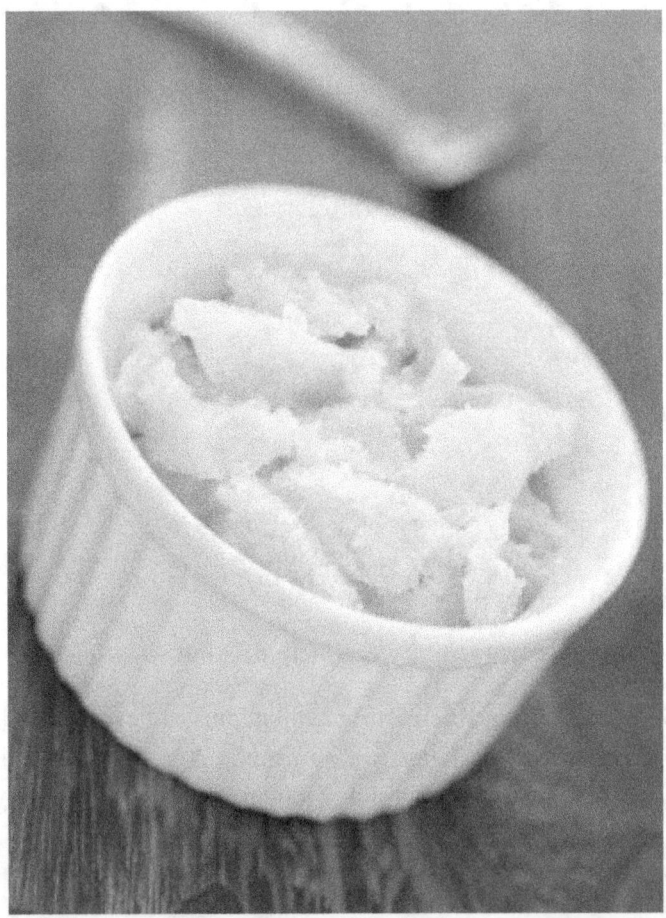

This is homemade butter, which has been heated, and is the most concentrated form of natural healthy oil available to you. If you buy it in the market, it is going to be exorbitantly priced. That is why it is much more sensible to make it at home.

Here is one good URL, where you can learn how to make ghee.

https://www.youtube.com/watch?v=SnXGhDugX7s.

In many parts of the East, this clarified butter has been used traditionally to make up many traditional medicines using dry fruit mixed with ghee.

In the same way, if you want to increase your energy level, all you need to do is take eight walnuts, six raisins, four almonds every day, early in the morning.

People in Asia feed their elders, eight walnuts, 4 almonds and 10 raisins every morning with a glassful of milk. This is their reason for good health, and good mental and physical strength even when the elders have reached their 80s and 90s. This can of course be eaten by young adults too, to keep healthy throughout their lives.

Or if you really want instant energy, that is done by taking 25 g of walnuts, fried in ghee and mixed with honey, according to taste, for one whole month. This is going to have a visible effect on your concentration power and your memory. We are not going to suffer from mental fatigue.

You could try eating five walnuts every day with meals. The best thing is, of course, to eat as many of these dry fruits as you can, and which you can digest without any problem to your system.

Walnut oil like almond oil can be used for massaging purposes. It is also an essential part of aromatherapy.

Walnuts for Skincare

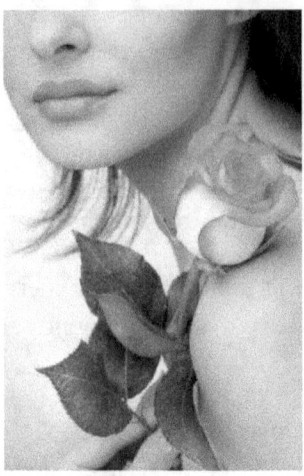

When I was a young child, living in an area which was not very salubrious because of a moist and fuggy atmosphere and Bad water, most of our friends and their parents were prone to boils, pimples and other skin infections. Not us though. That was because we were fed five walnuts by our grandmother, everyday with breakfast.

I do not know whether this was enough to keep our immunity system working well to prevent any sort of skin infection, but believe it or not, I have never suffered from any skin ailment brought about by bad water or by dirt, dust and grime. This includes boils, ringworm, and pimples.

She also advocated one good way in which one could cure ringworm. Five walnuts chewed properly, first thing in the morning – without washing out your mouth or brushing your teeth before hand – was good to cure ringworm. Along with that, a Walnut paste was applied on the affected area and within 10 days, you could see the fungal infection disappearing and the skin curing healthy and naturally.

This is because walnuts, like other dried fruit is considered to be an extremely good blood purifier. In olden days, people thought ringworm to be caused due to impure blood, along with pimples and other skin diseases. That is why wise old women knew that they needed human psychology in order to make people follow the elementary rules of hygiene.

The Magic of Walnuts

That is why they told them to wash in water in which these dry fruit like almonds, and walnuts had been soaked overnight. You ate the almonds and walnuts – you washed in its water. And you found a difference.

The difference was apparent and visible. You had washed the grime off your skin. So there was no chance of infection. Apart from that, you had eaten dry fruits, which were healthy, nourishing and nutritive. This strengthened your immunity system. A little bit of applied psychology, and there you were, cured due to a little bit of wisdom and a little bit of elementary hygiene, supported by knowledge about dry fruits!

Walnuts for Chest Infections

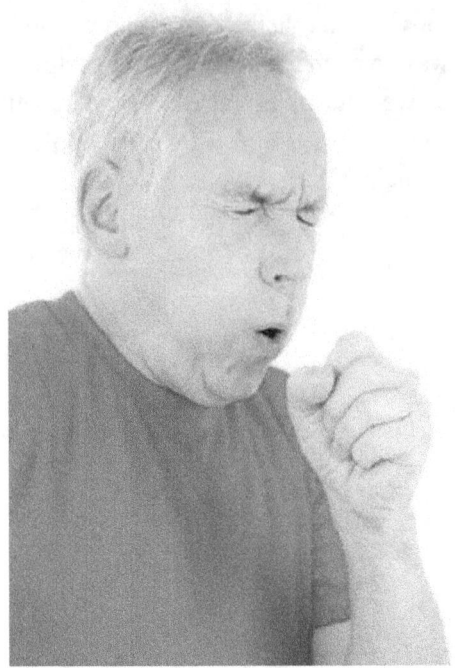

Walnuts have long been used for curing chest infections, especially if you are suffering from chronic cough and colds, or just infections brought about with the onset of winter.

Take five walnuts and fry them on the griddle. Eat them hot with a glassful of milk, last thing before you go off to sleep. If you are suffering from cough, in the winter, you may want to add a spoonful of Ghee during the frying process. This is going to keep you warm, and prevent any sort of infections.

In olden days, people suffered from TB, just because of the unhygienic conditions in which they lived. So people look for ways and means in which this could be prevented or cured or even stopped from proceeding any further.

For this, you needed eight walnuts and four cloves of garlic. These were then fried in ghee, and fed to the patient. This would bring about a marked improvement in the health of the patient.

Now here is the explanation. Walnuts give you natural strength. Garlic has long been considered to be a really good antiseptic and antiviral and antibacterial antibiotic in ancient and modern traditional medicine. It would help boost the immunity system along with ghee. So the patient's health would improve considerably. Elementary, my dear Watson.

Precautions and Possible Side Effects

Many people have complained of sores in their mouths, after eating walnuts. This could happen to anybody, especially if his system has developed some sort of allergy to one particular food item. This is the reason why so many people in the world today are suffering from gluten allergy. That is because the chemical pollutants in the atmosphere around them have affected their natural biochemical makeup in such a way that their natural ability to digest gluten has been impaired.

This is one trend which has started and it is going to continue throughout the years. You may find yourself not able to assimilate one particular food item, because your system rejects it.

So firstly, you need to stop eating that food and see if your system goes back to normal again. Then slowly start eating that food again in smaller quantities to make sure that your body gets accustomed to that particular intake of food in your normal day to day diet.

You can then slowly and steadily build up an increase in your food intake. This is the only way in which you can prevent future allergies from taking over your life.

So if you are suffering from a sore mouth after you have eaten walnuts, stop eating them for the next 4 – 5 days. Then eat a couple of walnuts, and see if the sores come back. If they do not, it means that you can tolerate a couple of walnuts with your daily meals. The next week, add just one more Walnut to your intake until you manage five, which should be adequate for one days' Omega-3 intake through walnuts.

Conclusion

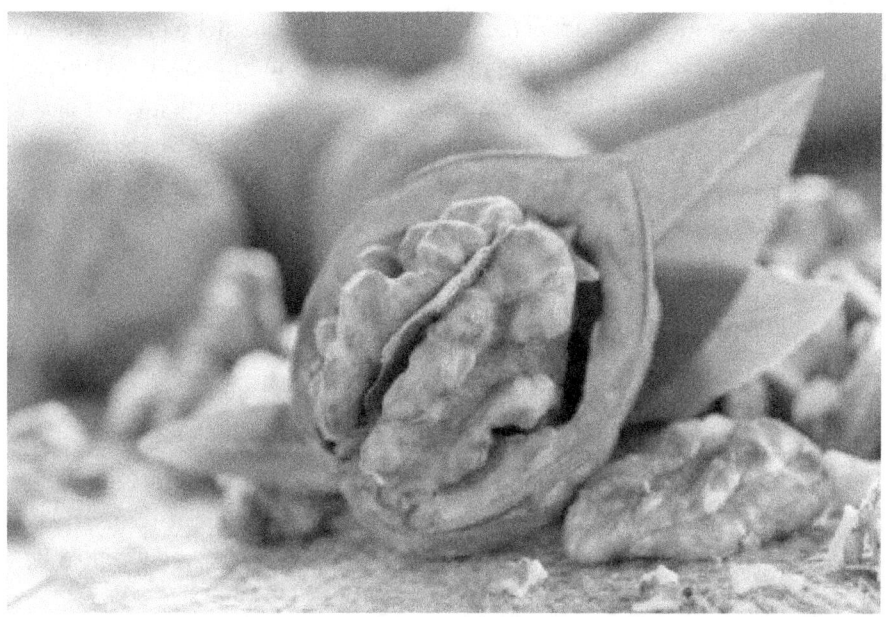

This book is going to give you an invaluable insight into the nutritive qualities of walnuts, along with other dried fruit, which are necessary to keep you healthy throughout your life.

Walnuts are considered to be extremely excellent brain food nuts. So adding them to your daily diet is going to enhance your memory and concentration power. This is necessary for a person who is more into brainwork than brawn work.

So take a handful of walnuts right away and get chewing. Add these nuts along with almonds, raisins and other easily available dry fruit to your daily diet right away. You are soon going to find a visible improvement in your health and find yourself working with renewed energy. That is the power of these nutritious, health giving and tasty nuts.

Live Long and Prosper!

Author Bio

Dueep Jyot Singh is a Management and IT Professional who managed to gather Postgraduate qualifications in Management and English and Degrees in Science, French and Education while pursuing different enjoyable career options like being an hospital administrator, IT,SEO and HRD Database Manager/ trainer, movie , radio and TV scriptwriter, theatre artiste and public speaker, lecturer in French, Marketing and Advertising, ex-Editor of Hearts On Fire (now known as Solstice) Books Missouri USA, advice columnist and cartoonist, publisher and Aviation School trainer, ex-moderator on Medico.in, banker, student councilor ,travelogue writer … among other things!

One fine morning, she decided that she had enough of killing herself by Degrees and went back to her first love -- writing. It's more enjoyable! She already has 48 published academic and 14 fiction- in- different- genre books under her belt.

When she is not designing websites or making Graphic design illustrations for clients , she is browsing through old bookshops hunting for treasures, of which she has an enviable collection – including R.L. Stevenson, O.Henry, Dornford Yates, Maurice Walsh, De Maupassant, Victor Hugo, Sapper, C.N. Williamson, "Bartimeus" and the crown of her collection- Dickens "The Old Curiosity Shop," and so on… Just call her "Renaissance Woman") - collecting herbal remedies, acting like Universal Helping Hand/Agony Aunt, or escaping to her dear mountains for a bit of exploring, collecting herbs and plants and trekking.

Check out some of the other JD-Biz Publishing books

Gardening Series on Amazon

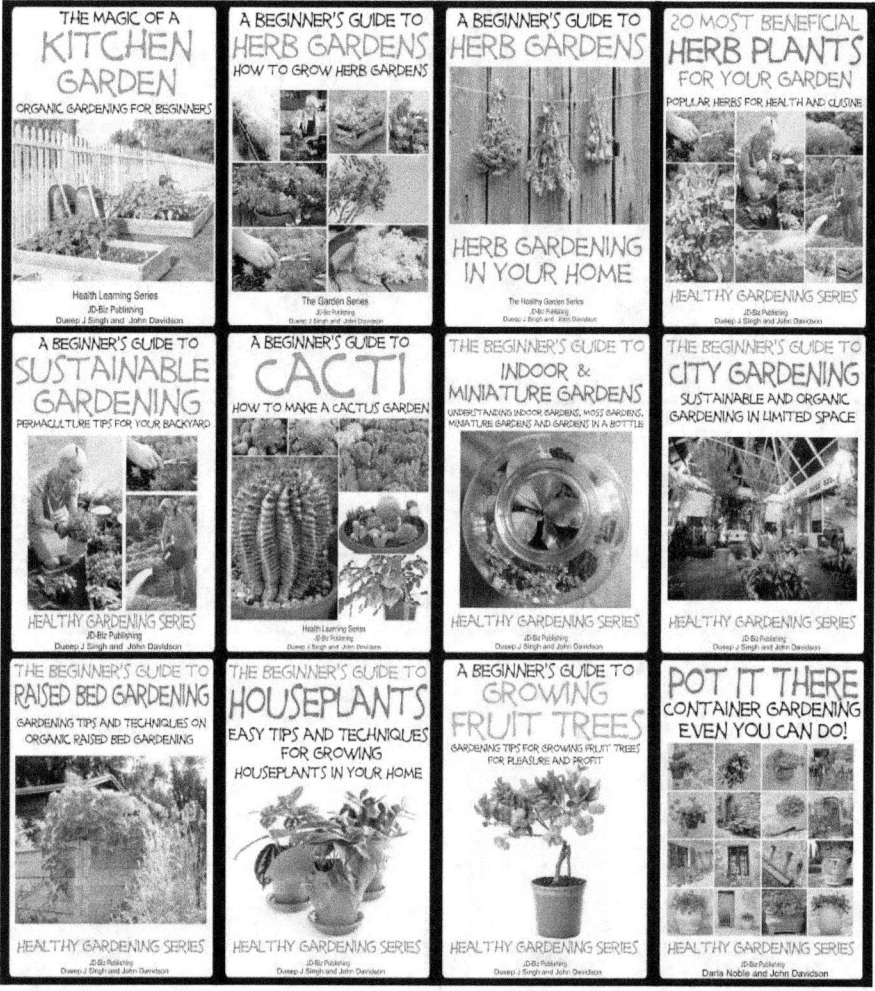

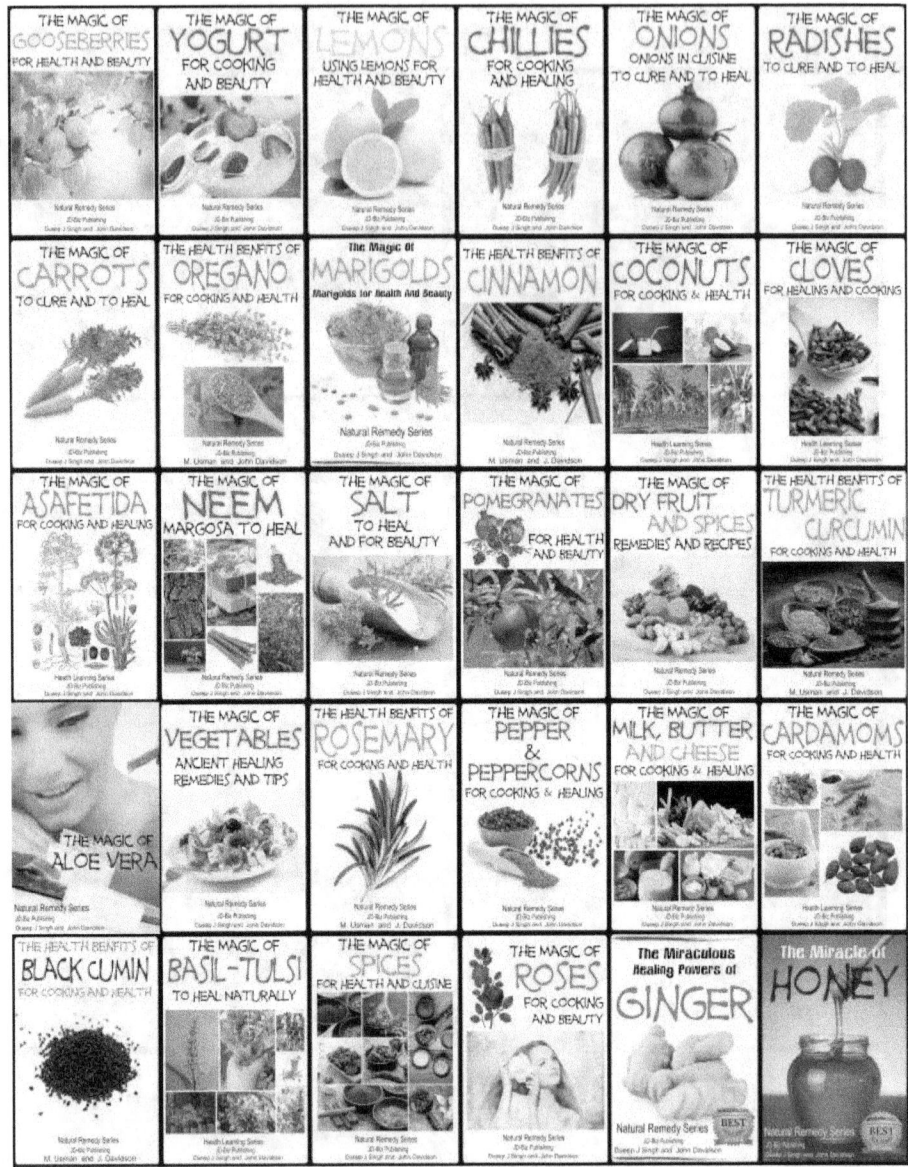

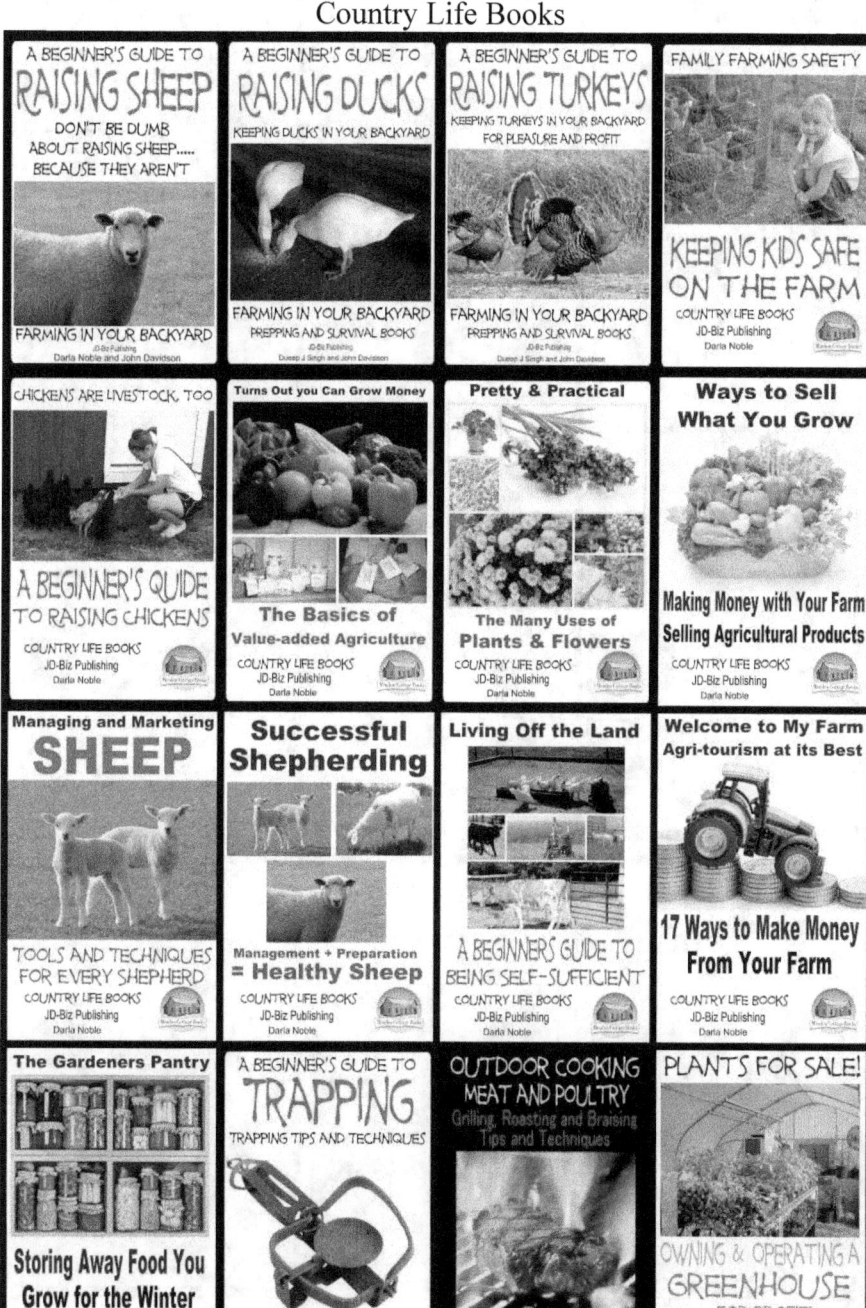

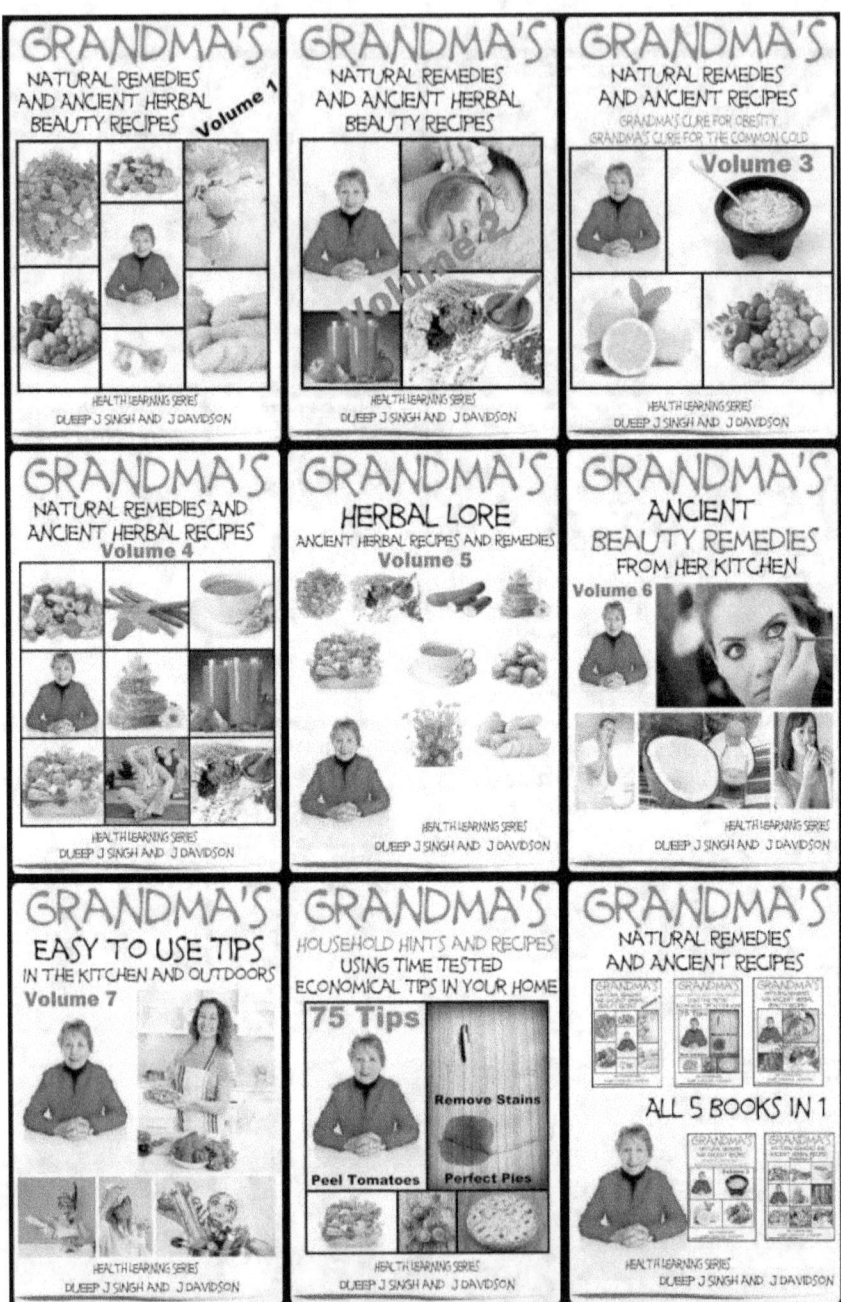

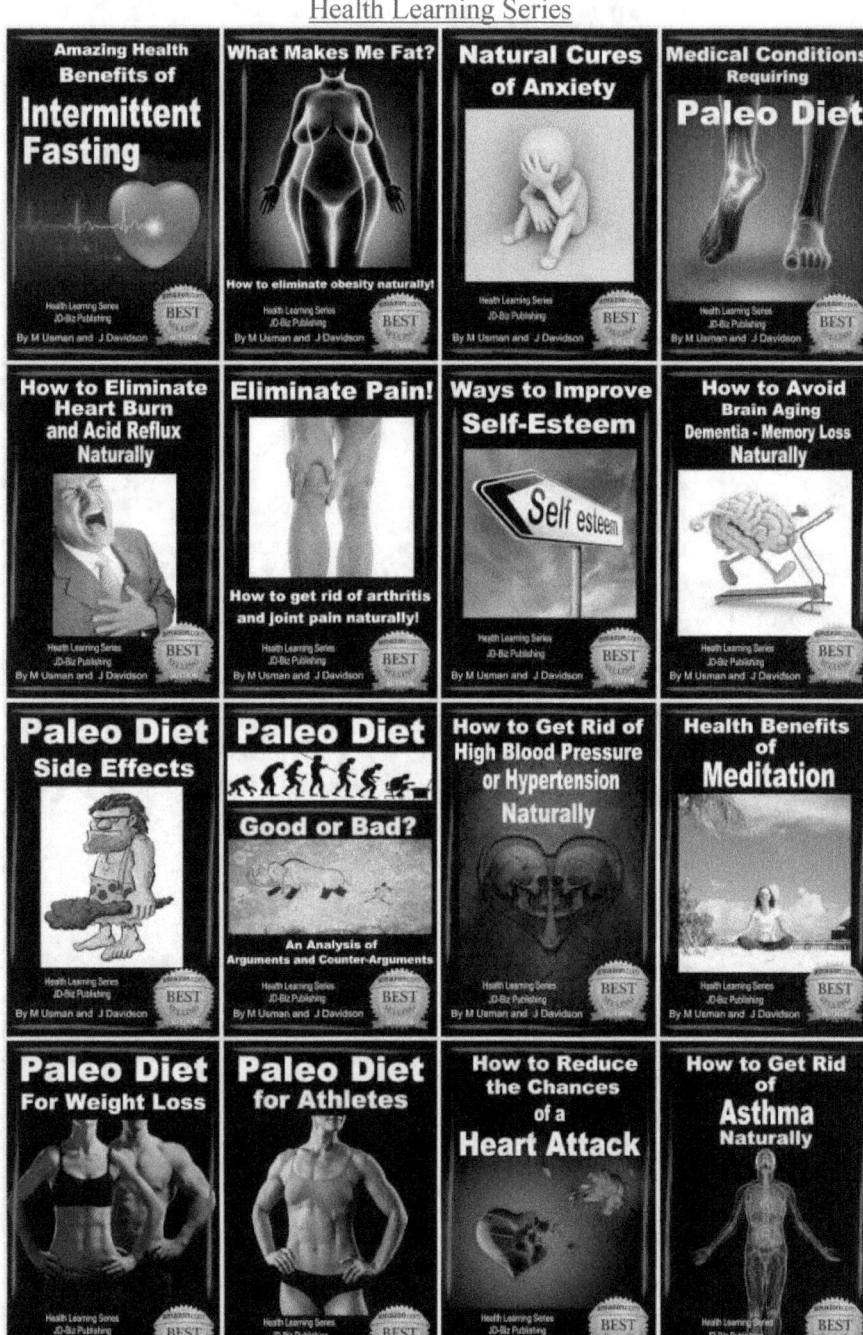

The Magic of Walnuts

Amazing Animal Book Series

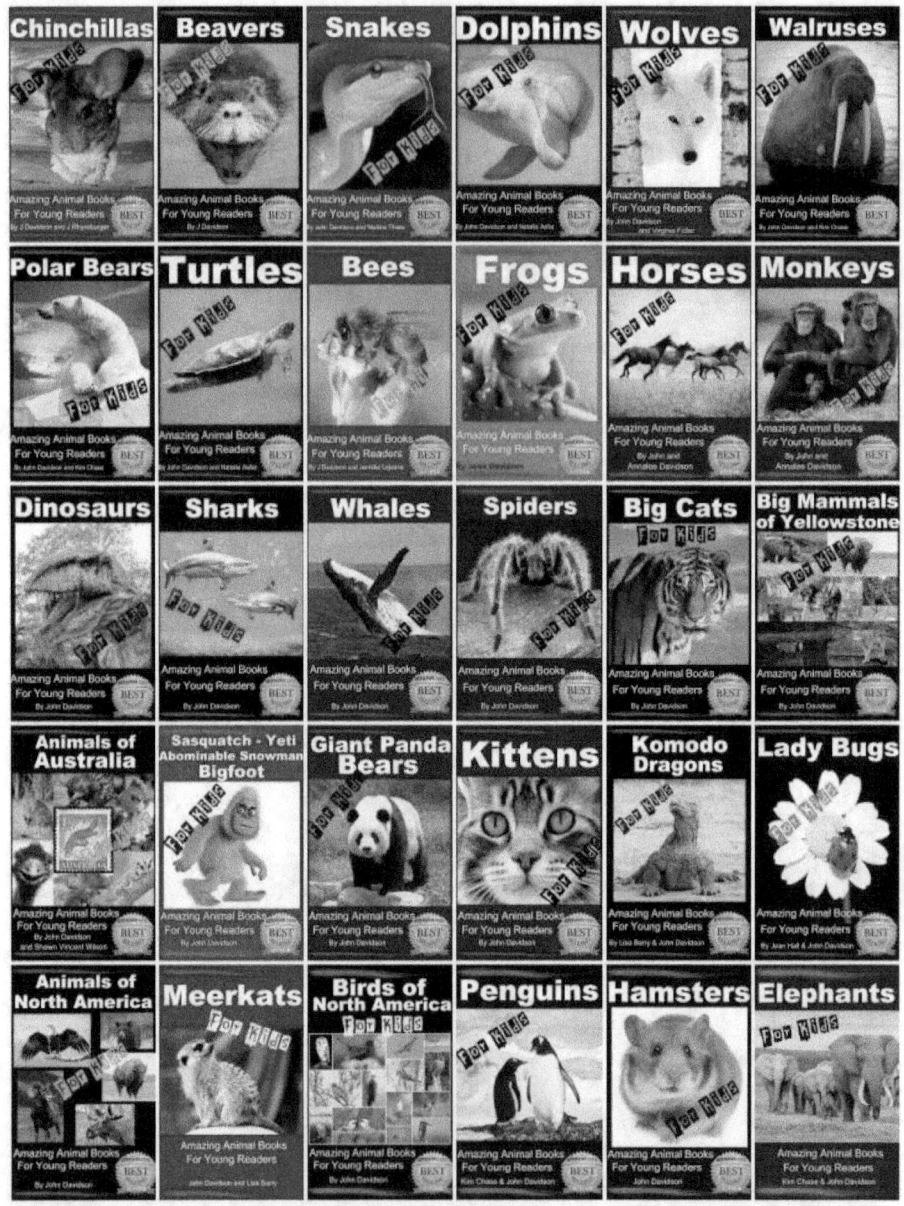

The Magic of Walnuts

Learn To Draw Series

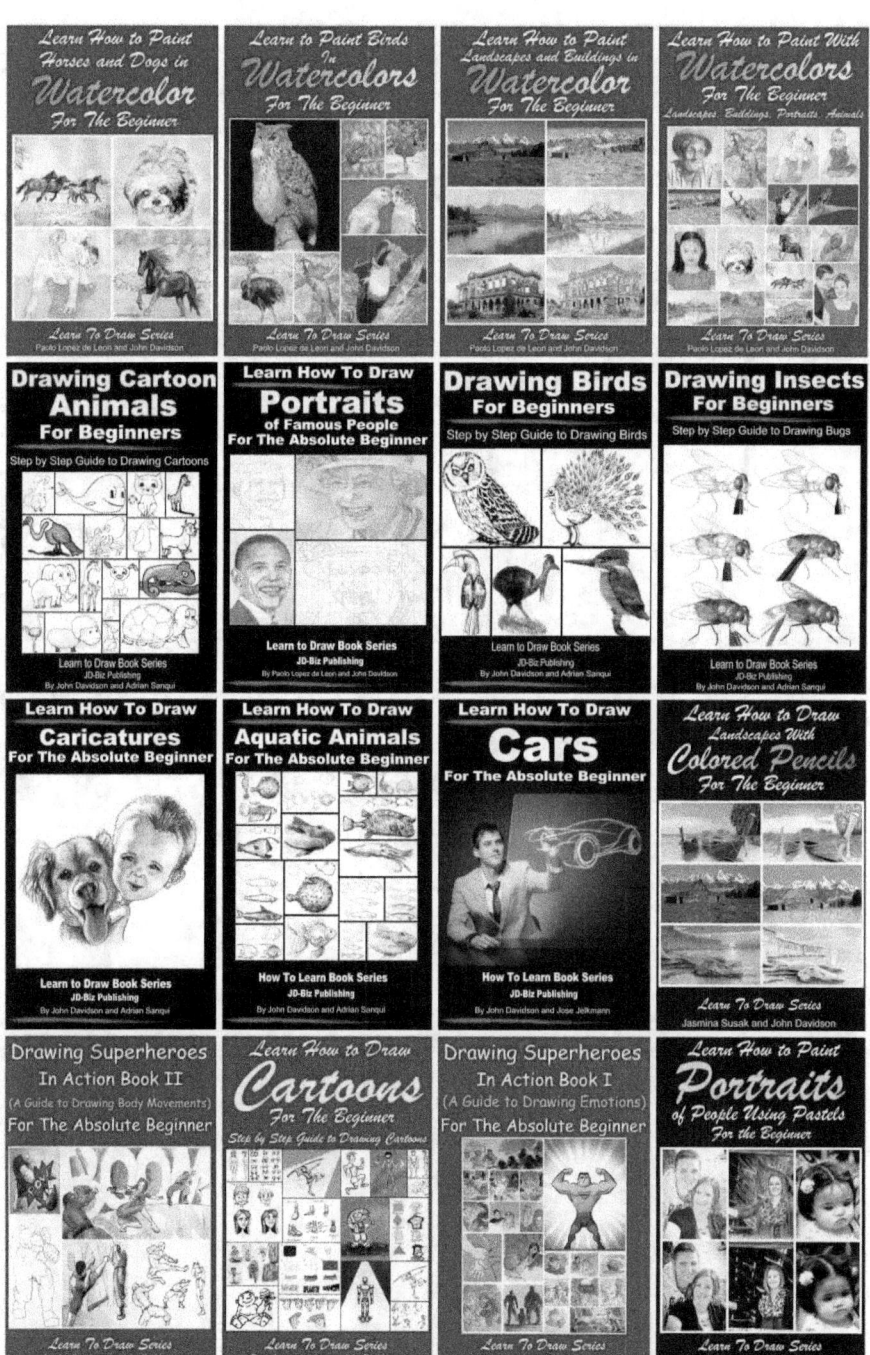

The Magic of Walnuts

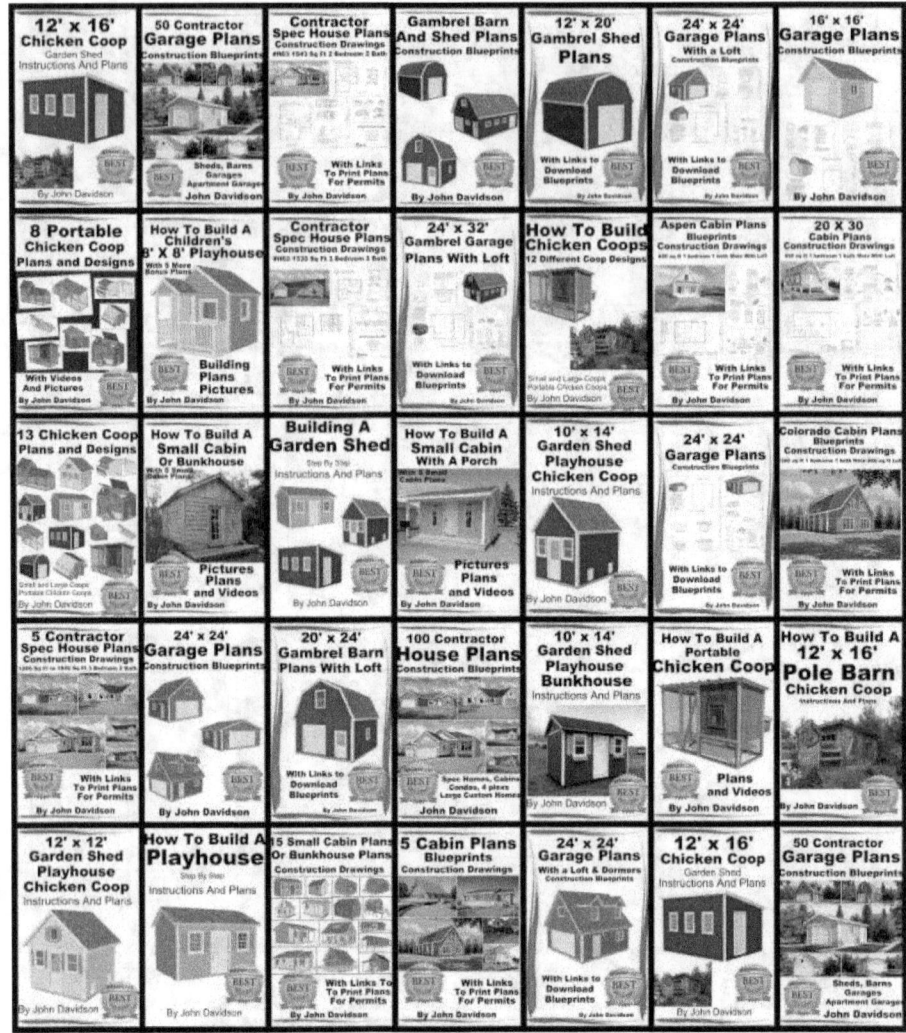

Entrepreneur Book Series

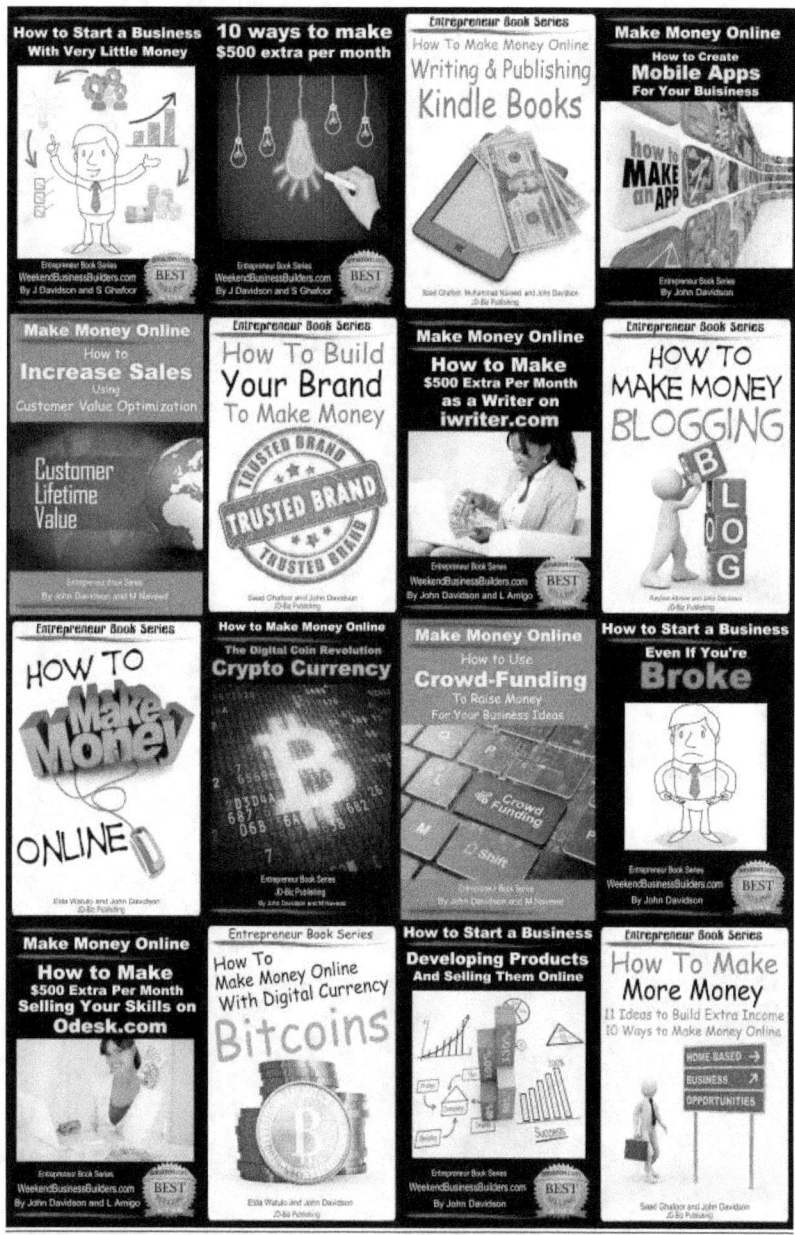

Our books are available at

1. Amazon.com

2. Barnes and Noble

3. Itunes

4. Kobo

5. Smashwords

6. Google Play Books

Publisher

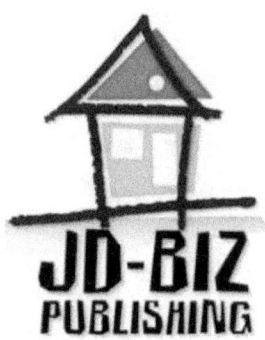

JD-Biz Corp

P O Box 374

Mendon, Utah 84325

http://www.jd-biz.com/

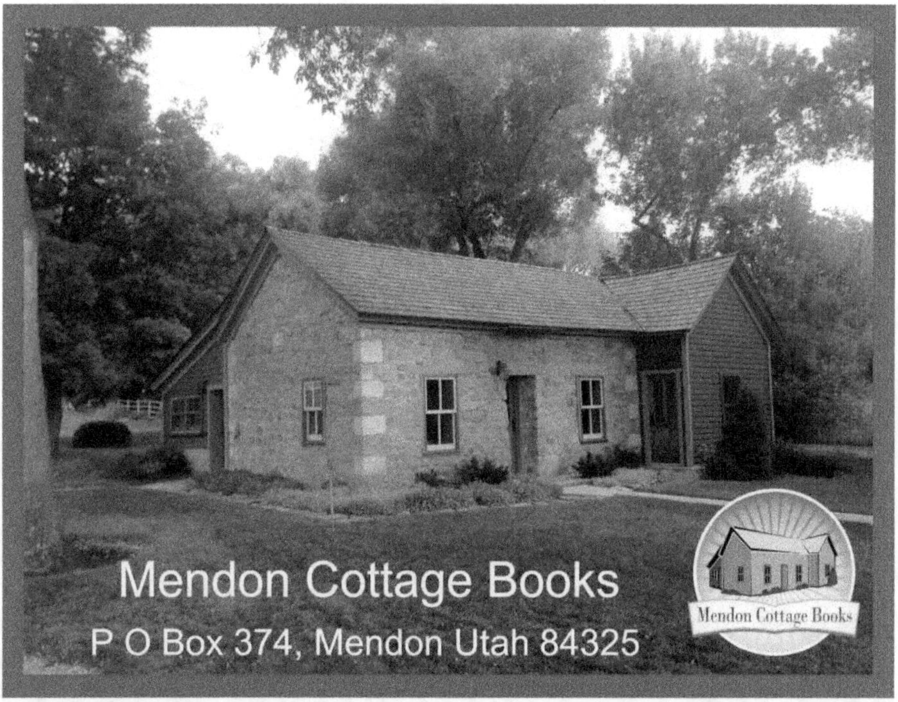

Mendon Cottage Books

P O Box 374, Mendon Utah 84325

The Magic of Walnuts

www.ingramcontent.com/pod-product-compliance
Lightning Source LLC
Chambersburg PA
CBHW061804280526
45787CB00003BA/1473